MW00908832

ALKALINE LIFESTYLE AND HOLISTIC NUTRITION TIPS FOR MODERN PEOPLE

By Marta Tuchowska

Copyright © 2014, 2015 Marta Tuchowska

www.HolisticWellnessProject.com

www.AlkalineDietLifestyle.com

The book is not intended to provide medical advice or to take the place of medical advice and treatment from your personal physician. Readers are advised to consult their own doctors or other qualified health professionals regarding the treatment of medical conditions. The author shall not be held liable or responsible for any misunderstanding or misuse of the information contained in this book. The information is not intended to diagnose, treat or cure any disease.

It is important to remember that the author of this book is not a doctor/ medical professional. Only opinions based upon her own personal experiences or research are cited. THE AUTHOR DOES NOT OFFER MEDICAL ADVICE or prescribe any treatments. For any health or medical issues – you should be talking to your doctor first.

Alkaline Diet Motivation

INTRODUCTION All you need to understand to achieve massive "alkaline" success...5

PART I: MOTIVATION All you need to know about mindful eating. Have your holistic health and wellness vision and stick to it...10

PART II: ALKALINE MINDSET Are you ready to invest in your health and wellness success? If not, why not?...12

PART III: PREPARATION Success is yours if you are willing to take it!...19

PART IV: ALKALINE AND HOLISTIC NUTRITION TIPS Understanding the basics of the Alkaline Diet and making it your lifestyle. "Lifestyle" sounds better than a "diet", right?...30

PART V: BONUS CHAPTER – 20+ EASY ALKALINE RECIPES How to embrace Alkalinity!...57

INTRODUCTION

WHY I WROTE THIS BOOK

So many of my friends and clients get interested in the Alkaline Diet and want to give it a shot. It's enough to have a look at weight loss, health and wellness benefits that it offers. The first reaction is usually: "Yes, I want to try it! Sounds great!" Unfortunately, many people give up; many of them say it is too difficult to do the Alkaline Diet. Now, I am not here to tell you that it's super easy, but I can assure you that once you organize yourself and apply certain rules and make them your lifestyle, it will become automatic. And yes, it will become easy for you. If you want to get committed to *alkaline wellness*, you have come to the right place. I am here to show you how you can make it easier and how you can alkalize your body and mind and have fun while doing so.

"Great changes may not happen right away, but with effort, even the difficult may become easy." Bill Blackma

The way I put it is: *Failure is easier than success. So, do you really want to take the easy route?*

This is why I have written this book. It is a quick guide of different "alkaline" tips related to:
- balanced nutrition in general (in my opinion, Alkaline Diet is about seeking balance)
- mind and body wellness- balanced nutrition is not only about weight loss, it is also about feeling amazing in your body, being able to focus and control YOUR emotions. This is what I call *Holistic Wellness*. If you want to embark on your journey of self-development you must commit yourself to healthy nutrition. Proper self-care is a must. Unfortunately, in this day and age it is also a big challenge for many people.

5

- <u>What to add and what do avoid</u>- when you already eat healthy and alkaline, you usually develop this amazing natural ability to listen to your body. For example, now I know when I need to add more super alkaline foods to my diet (my energy levels tell me). I also know when it's OK, to have some neutral or slightly acidic foods. I know how to find balance, but when you first get started on the Alkaline Diet (or healthy eating in general) it is good to have some clear guidelines. Then, the more you "alkalize", the better you feel and so you want to carry on your alkaline journey.

- <u>Preparation tips</u>- people often blame lack of time, which I can understand. I have been there many times myself. However, if you put some effort now and learn a few alkaline tricks, you will be able to save your precious time later. It's all about developing a system. I am a big fan of developing systems that help me improve different areas of my life and systems are also great if you want to take care of your health and fitness. In other words, you may have to toughen up a bit and leave your comfort zone. It's easy to pick some ready-to-eat garbage foods, but *health success* is not about doing things that are easy. You need to learn how to be in charge of what you feed your body (and your mind) with. It all comes down to developing some new useful skills, that down the road you can always pass on to other people. You can teach your kids, family and friends. Health can be mastered. I am here to help you.

- Motivation tips- I want you to keep on track. I want you to be a *health and wellness warrior*. I also want you to become your own holistic health coach. Reading this book alone will not act as a magic procrastination cure. All I am asking you is to do at least a few days' challenge (a week's challenge would be even better!) to eat healthy and alkaline. I can't do it for you. Even if I could, I wouldn't do it. I want you to experience this amazing feeling of overcoming certain unhealthy habits

YOURSELF. I believe in you and I know that since you took an interest in this book (it's a mix of health and personal development), you will succeed. After that, your body will feel better and you will forget about "the mental fogginess" feeling. As you start experiencing more and more benefits of Alkalinity, it will become your lifestyle. If you feel good, why quit feeling good? There is no point in quitting, right?

I always say that ever since I turned to Alkalinity my creativity has improved. Other *alkalarians* I know, say exactly the same. Something has changed, not only on a physical level, but also on a mental level. I say "thanks" to the Alkaline Diet. Before discovering the alkaline diet I struggled with depression and no zest for life. I didn't know what to do. Alkalinity and Holistic Nutrition helped me start a new chapter in my life. A better one, a stronger one. Moreover, I was able to stop "dieting" and "calorie counting" and began to enjoy my new strong body and real physical fitness. I go to the gym every day and I train harder every day. I am loving it. <u>If I could do it, you can do it too.</u>

- BONUS CHAPTER- there are quite a few alkaline recipes included. They are designed for busy people and can help you switch to healthier alternatives. I hope they will stimulate your creativity and expand your cooking horizons.

Never heard of the Alkaline Diet and don't know where to start?

I remember when I first learned about the alkaline diet. I was more than confused and skeptical. I wanted to take action but didn't know how. I would spend endless hours online looking for alkaline-acid charts only to find there was way too much contradictory information out there.

7

I don't want you to feel confused. I also really appreciate the fact you took an interest in my work. This is why I would love to offer you a free, complimentary 100 page e-book and **easy alkaline-acid charts** (printable so that you can keep them on your fridge or in your wallet). It will provide a solid foundation to kick-start your alkaline diet success. You will get all the facts explained in plain English, practical alkaline tips, and yummy, vegan-friendly recipes full of taste, motivational advice, as well as printable charts for quick reference. I will also show you how to combine the alkaline lifestyle with other diets (Paleo, vegetarian, vegan). The alkaline diet is very flexible, and it always welcome all kinds of "Alkalarians." You don't have to be 100% vegan to follow an alkaline diet, the choice is always yours.

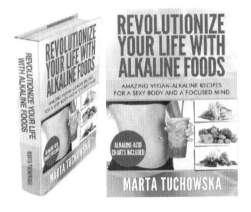

To download this eBook, please visit:

www.bitly.com/AlkalineMarta

or: www.holisticwellnessproject.com/alkaline-diet-ebook/giveaway.html

Alkaline Diet Motivation- The Real Deal

Health success is not only about knowing "stuff" and recipes, but also about applying them and making progress. I always say that there is information, motivation and inspiration. This book focuses mostly on motivation and inspiration. Many health professionals just stick with information and I personally think it's not enough if you want to be super successful. Motivational factor is of paramount importance my friend. We want visible results, right? A sexy body, focused mind and high energy levels- sound good?

*This book can be also helpful for those who are not really interested in the Alkaline Diet but are looking for quick tips to improve their general wellbeing and increase their energy levels;

*No matter which diet you have chosen to follow you can combine it with some of my tips included in this book. Take care of your health and help your family do the same;

*Maybe you are not new to Alkalinity, but you have gotten off track and need some motivational "refresher". I am sure this read will help you.

BUT, FIRST OF ALL...

*This book is a quick reference for those who are pressed for time and want to take care of their nutrition in a holistic way.

PART I: ALKALINE MOTIVATION

MINDFULNESS, AWARNESS AND HOLISTIC NUTRITION

Conscious eating is a step by step process in which you have ultimate control over the what, where, when, and how. When tackling an obstacle and striving for a goal it is important to remember that dedication is not measured by choice. It is an inherent and intangible aspect of our will, determination, commitment, and perseverance.

When choosing certain foods ask yourself this question:

"Does this meal bring me closer to my goals, or is it actually preventing me from achieving my health, weight loss and wellness success?"

Remember that society tricks us into something. We are told that everything is so easy and that "the faster the better". The result is our unhealthy and very often overweight generation that lacks knowledge and has no idea how to turn this situation around. This is a great selling market for not only medications (many diseases can be prevented or at least reduced by healthy nutrition), but also miracle weight loss pills, weight loss programs, and plenty of other just "newly discovered miraculous products". Don't waste your money, time and effort on quick *cures* that don't work.

What I have chosen for myself is to be mindful about what I eat. I want to invest in my future. I enjoy every second spent on healthy shopping and cooking. By doing things myself I know I am in charge. It is such a fantastic feeling that I want you to experience.

Be in charge. You deserve it.

I love mindful eating and mindful cooking. I no longer feel this disempowering need of watching TV and indulging in unhealthy foods. TV and foods that are poison go hand in hand together. In fact, TV is acidic! Most of the stuff that you watch is acidic for your mind. TV was designed to brainwash millions of people by its very nature. TV commercials are supposed to act on your subconscious mind and make you crave even more processed foods. Now, I have something better. If you are into mindful eating and cooking, here's my tip for you.

I treat time spent in the kitchen as relaxation or learning time. I plan and cook my meals and relax my mind and soul with some soothing ambient music. I may sometimes go for something more energetic, why not? Energetic beats set me for action and preparing my gym bag. I also use my cooking time to listen to some motivational podcasts and videos

Try it yourself and let me know what you think. Create your cooking and eating rituals. Imagine your kitchen is your holistic health spa.

Of course, there is nothing wrong about watching TV in moderation. I am not saying you have to stop watching TV forever. It's great to watch something you enjoy so that you can relax, laugh or learn something new. The problem is when we watch TV to escape from reality or simply kill time and we don't even know why we are watching it. Do you agree?

PART II: ALKALINE MINDSET

ALKALINE DIET: THE CONCEPT OF AN INVESTOR AND A CONSUMER

Remember: you are an investor, not a consumer. You analyze your choices and you think about your future. If you are a parent, your additional motivation should be getting new skills that you can pass onto your kids. You can teach them how to eat healthy. I was really lucky that my parents were into healthy eating and we ate pretty healthy (yes, pretty healthy as there was no fast-food). As a kid, I wanted to have some foods that my peers were having (*forbidden fruit!*) and I would just tell my parents:

" ....*but everyone is eating this or that, or everyone is buying this or that, or everyone is having this for breakfast/lunch at school*".

Luckily, both my dad and my mom would just tell me:

"You *don't want to be like everyone else*".

Throughout my childhood and teenage years, I very often struggled because I wanted to be like everyone else. Now I am happy and proud of the healthy education that my parents gave me. I am also proud of the fact that I am not like everyone else. My tip for you- when you start your healthy eating lifestyle, you may be different than those around you. Simply embrace this feeling. As Mark Twain said (I am paraphrasing):

"*If you are in the majority, then it's time to change it as you have a big problem...*"

Maybe this is not your case. Maybe you were born in a family where nobody paid attention to healthy eating and obesity was "something normal". Some say that obesity is genetic. I agree that genes play an important part in the way our body is. However, don't use it as an excuse. "Fat" genes should be an alarm that is telling you to take action and take even better care of yourself. This means that you may have it a bit harder than other people who are lucky enough to have "slim genes". Accept it and don't use it as an excuse. There is always someone who has had it easier than you and someone who has had it harder than you.

For example...Your neighbor may be born with "slim genes" and is abusing his/her body with processed foods and empty calories. Eventually they will put on weight and may get some serious health condition. You may be born with "fat genes", but you accept it. This should motivate you to eat healthy and exercise. You may be slimmer and healthier than those who have "slim genes", but lack character and perseverance.

I know lots of people who grew up on fast food. It is not that their families didn't care, it's just that their families <u>didn't know</u> what they were doing. They were simply following everyone else. Now, it is time for you to break this vicious cycle. You can learn the basics of healthy, holistic nutrition and help your family. You can educate yourself and make sure that your kids have it easier. You know I believe in you. You know you are on the right track. Your moment of triumph is very close...

Let me put it this way: you have some kind of responsibility here my friend. If you don't take action someone out there may not get exposed to your healthy example and influence. Someone from your family or friends may be going to bed feeling sad, lacking energy and even overweight. Someone might be even losing hope. This is why you can't chicken out now. You are in my club! No turning back.

If you try to change something yourself you will be happy. As I said, my family did take care about healthy nutrition, but I have friends whose parents were even healthier than mine.

However, there were some things that I did not get taught at home; my parents were not at all into sports, they did not like physical activity at all. I used to be jealous of kids whose parents would teach them sports and encourage them to be physically active. As a kid I would always be horrible at PE class. However, when I was a teenager I decided to change it. I went for a high water jump- me and one of my high school friends, found local kick boxing classes and started training. We were the only girls in class and so we could not complain about lack of help. Those guys always wanted to help us. Moreover, the level of training was "pretty masculine" and so we both had to toughen up and keep up with it in order to get stronger.

The moment my parents saw my new "fitness" lifestyle and how it changed my self-esteem and even my performance in school and my ability to focus, they decided to take on sports as well. Lesson learned, even if you were not taught something, you can change it. Plus you can be a *living example* and help those around you change as well.

What I want you to understand is that you need to make a choice. Yes, right now! Some of your friends may tell you that you are weird or that you are too concerned about your health or that you exaggerate. Don't let them stop you; make it your mission to carry on. What you do, should serve as an example to other people. Just keep going. You are a health warrior!

Naturally, some days will be better than others, but eventually your conscious eating choices will become unconscious decisions based solely on the quality of the output it leads to. Eventually, you will constantly be seeking out the things that make you feel great and perform at your best; and it will be second nature to you. <u>This is alkaline success that I want you to achieve.</u>

When I first tried the alkaline diet, I found it hard to "synchronize" my eating habits with my partner's. He wasn't really interested in Alkalinity. I would just preach to him and this would make things worse. My boyfriend hates being told what to do, fair enough, I am the same. The worst thing is to do things because you have to, not because you want to. You must admit I am making a good point here, right?

This is why I simply decided to shut up and gave him a break. I decided to explore the art of healthy alkaline cooking and came up with a myriad of delicious alkaline recipes that he became a big fan of. He was surprised when I told him: "You have just had a super healthy alkaline dinner". The thing is that he associated Alkalinity with pain, he thought that it was a "rabbit's diet" or some green smoothie fad. And then, he found himself eating alkaline meals and really enjoying them. I taught him that Alkalinity is more about achieving balance. Even if you are a carnivorous animal, or your eating tendencies are focused on diets like the Paleo diet (which, by the way is not only about eating massive amounts of meat, Paleo people also eat veggies, fruits, nuts and seeds), you can still add more alkaline foods to your diet and restore the energy levels. The Alkaline Diet will help you reduce meat and dairy as it is full of other, healthier and tastier options. You don't have to go strictly vegan/vegetarian unless you want to (this is topic for another book).

The Alkaline Diet is really flexible.

Many popular fad diets will have you believe that dietary success is only achieved if your food will completely match their food agenda. Have this for breakfast, count calories, wait and repeat. By the way, I am not against counties calories, but from my experience counting calories took my *emotional wellness* away at some point. This made it difficult to get it back. What works for me is focusing on wholesome, alkaline, nourishing foods and trying not to get too paranoid about calorie counting. If I keep it that way I know that my body and mind are balanced so I don't crave for unhealthy garbage foods. Since I feel well-fed, I am not prone to binge-eating or other temptations.

INDIVIDUALITY AND HOLISTIC APPROACH

But what works for one might not work for another. I always say that I am not telling you what to do. I am telling you what I do. The last thing I want to become is a preaching guru. I want to provide you with inspiration and information so that you can create your own *alkaline wellness*.

The Alkaline Diet respects and encourages individuality. The intent of this book is self-empowerment. With this book I strive to provide you with knowledge. For example, tools to make healthy choices that will compliment your bodies systems through better, more efficient metabolism. This is what I call sustainable weight-loss. You make conscious choices today and you will be reaping off multiple health and weight loss benefits tomorrow, next week, and years to come.

Listen to your body, observe, compare and team up with it. You and your body are like a team!

Over the past hundred years our diets have undergone some major changes, this is especially true for the Western world. Consequently, the majority of us have some form (or forms for some) of mineral deficiency. Therefore, for our own well-being it is vital that we make better food choices. We all know the basic benefits of eating right. For example, weight loss, a

16

strong immune system, increased energy and stamina. Though the right combinations of food along with a complete and efficient system of metabolism and digestion can give you all of that, plus:

1. mental clarity and increased cognitive functioning
2. longer, deeper sleeping
3. better respiratory functioning , deeper breathing
4. increased sex drive

TREAT YOURSELF WITH HEALTH. YOU DESERVE THE BEST!

Creating a healthy lifestyle is exciting and fun, just follow these steps:

- ***Write your intent.*** You've heard of food journaling where you write down everything that you eat in a day? Well, let the preface be your mission statement. State in your most honest and sincerest words why this is so important to you and what you wish to achieve. Will you be making yourself get up early to exercise? Why? Tell the book all about it. Don't be shy or holdback on details or insight into feelings or motives. Remember that ultimately this is for you and your benefit. Why start incomplete and withholding? I mean, how long can you afford to wait? I suggest you start planning your month, then chunk it down and plan each week and day. If you are new to planning you may want to start planning your week first. Then focus on every day. Make it your mission and be passionate about it.

- **Set realistic goals/benchmarks.** End the vicious cycle once and for all. You know the one where you get all pumped up, swear that you're going to "do it this time". Completely turn your daily routine upside down with calorie counting and exercising, only to 'see' nothing happen after all the hard work. Estimates say that the average dieter expects a quick turn-around time with a loss of 50% of their problem weight. Most diets are deemed failures and abandoned in less than 6 weeks.

Another thing about "dieting" is that "dieters" often see their diet as something painful and temporary. Even if they finish their "program", healthy eating is not their habit and so quite naturally their brain sabotages them and they get back right to where they were before

One more thing...the Alkaline Diet is not just a diet. Let's call it a lifestyle, or the alkaline diet lifestyle, ok? Let's forget about "eliminating". Let's focus on adding, energizing and alkalizing. Yes! Let's keep adding plenty of fresh veggies and other alkaline foods. We need energy that will help us achieve massive wellness success.

Mini exercise for you: what can you add now, today? Maybe one big raw salad a day? Maybe a big glass of fresh veggie juice or a smoothie? Maybe, you can get some natural, alkaline supplements like alfalfa or liquid chlorophyll? Drink more clean water?
Maybe you can add more physical activity? What is your plan? Choose one thing and stick to it. Then, keep adding more.

PART III PREPARATION

Let's go through the tools that will ensure 'you will get there'.

- ***Change its name.*** *This is something I have just pointed to when talking about "dieting" and "dieters".* We all hold preconceived notions, definitions and expectations that determine our attitudes towards health. This is a natural process for the body to prepare us for upcoming situations. Subsequently, past experiences pre-orient, undermine perspective, and steal motivation. Thus, don't refer to it as a diet; call it a *healthy lifestyle* or something similar. Your new healthy lifestyle is fun, creative and exciting. Don't feed your mind with anything else, unless you want to make it harder for yourself...

- ***Banish those foods!*** Half-eaten bags of chips or cookies, unopened cans of beer or soda all represent temptations. So rid yourself and your house from them. Remove every morsel, crumb, or tantalizing drop of what might bring you doubt or 'ideas'. Out of sight out of mind- surround yourself with healthy foods that you deserve! If you really love snacking and chips, simply make them natural and alkaline. Check out this recipe:

Kale Chips

Kale chips, also called kale crisps in some English-speaking countries, are my favorite non-guilty pleasure. They are so delicious and addicting. I love that I can eat as many as I like to curb my cravings, while getting extra vitamins into my daily diet. They are easy to make and delicious.

1. Rinse one or two bunches of kale and allow drying.

2. Rip your kale into bite sized pieces.

3. Drizzle kale with about one tablespoon of oil for each bunch in a large bowl. Massage the leaves and get oil into all of the nooks and crannies. Season well to your liking.

4. Preheat oven to 300 degrees Fahrenheit or 145 Celsius, and bake for 10-12 minutes. When it is stiff and crispy with browned edges, remove immediately from the oven. Eat when cool.

- ***Protein***
  Contrary to the common belief protein is available in many vegetables and not just in meat. Somewhere, we gained the overriding belief that the heaviest and most un-nutritious foods provide the most 'fuel' for our bodies. Keep lite and healthy fruits and veggies around. Food such as celery sticks or carrot sticks provide ample protein. Natural organic yogurts, quinoa and nuts are also good sources. If you combine integral rice (can be also millet, amaranth and quinoa) with legumes (for example lentils, chickpeas and adzuki) you will obtain a natural and healthy source of protein. Now, legumes are not that alkaline, but they are much less acidic than meat. Meat is not the only source of protein and natural integral grains and legumes are not bad for you, as long as they are eaten in moderation and organic. Test what works for you. For example, I like to cook lentils and

freeze them in small portions and then use them for my salads (I usually add only a few tablespoons of lentils). My digestive system finds it difficult to digest large amounts of legumes, but small portions are fine.

- If you are Paleo, remember to add as many super alkaline foods to your diet as possible. Treat yourself to a big bowl of salad before your main course. Serve your meat on big heaps of salads and veggies. Here's the list of the most alkaline-forming foods ever:

        -Broccoli
        -Cucumber
        -Kale
        -Kelp
        -Soy Sprouts and Alfalfa Sprouts
        -Sea vegetables
        -Green Drinks
        -Sprouts
        -Spinach (baby and grown)
        -Parsley
        -Lemons (yes, they are alkaline!)
        -Herbs
        -Avocados
        -Tomatoes
        -Radishes
        -Almonds and Almond Milk
        -Garlic

- ***Bored or hungry?***
It seems that quantity is heavily regarded over quality. Remember, it's not about eating less but about eating right. We also need to practice awareness. Do we eat because we need to fuel our body? Or maybe because we are bored or stressed out?

It's a good bet that we will end up consuming unhealthy, chemical and additive laden starch based convenience food. Solution? Add more alkaline smoothies and healthy snacks like nuts and seeds into your diet. They will help you feel nicely energized and nourished.

- ***Be particularly mindful of those unhealthy snacks.***
  If you want to snack, go for it. Just opt for the less demanding and lighter foods, such as a piece of fruit. Have a glass of warm almond milk (choose the natural, raw one). Almond milk is really alkalizing and will give you a nice comfort sensation. You can add some barley grass powder for optimal nutrition. A tablespoon of coconut oil can also help you fight sugar cravings. It will help you sleep better and satisfy your sweet tooth. If you think that your urge to do some nighttime snacking is emotional (most of these are emotional, in my opinion) and the root of the problem is stress, I suggest you switch to aromatherapy instead. Treat is as a ritual. You can learn more from my book: "Essential Oils for Weight Loss". You can find it on my blog: www.HolisticWellnessProject.com in the "books" section.

Aromatherapy is Alkaline. It forms part of the alkaline lifestyle and not only does it soothe and relax your body and mind, but it helps you avoid artificial skin products. Skin is the largest human organ. If you use artificial body lotions and creams, you make even more toxins enter your body and create more acidity.

My blog also features several articles that will help your create your aromatherapy home spa and prevent emotional night time snacking.

For extra information, check out:
www.holisticwellnessproject.com/blog/natural-therapy-spa

Let me give you a few of my aromatherapy tricks that will help you relax, prevent insomnia and emotional eating, I recommend this ritual at night time:

- Choose 1 to 3 of the following essential oils: lavender, verbena, bergamot, mandarin, sweet orange, and palmarosa.
- Mix about 6 drops (in total, if you are using more than 1 essential oil) in 1 tablespoon of vegetable base oil (it can be coconut oil, sweet almond oil, grape seed oil or any other oil of your choice as long as it is natural, organic and cold pressed).
- Massage your neck, arms and solar plexus. Breathe in and out. Enjoy the moment.
- I also recommend 2 drops of chamomile essential oil mixed with 2 drops of lavender essential oil diluted in 1 tablespoon of your chosen vegetable oil. Massage your face and neck, paying attention to your forehead. If you have really sensitive skin, test this blend on your arm first, but chamomile and lavender are really save oils and normally suitable for sensitive complexions (like mine).

This was the basic piece of information that even the busiest modern individual can apply to relax and unwind. Alkaline Lifestyle is not only about what you eat, it's also about how you live...Holistic Relaxation is something that can be learned.

- **Learn the power of sleep.** Sleeping produces two hormones, ghrelin and leptin. The former activates the hunger signal while the latter signals enough or full. Under sleeping suppresses leptin causing us to perceive the inability to get full. 6- 8 hours of sleep is the standard recommendation, naturally yours might differ to accommodate illness or other disorders. Recent studies reveal that the consequences of not getting adequate sleep are a lot more damaging and touch on more are thought. Lack of sleep can adversely affect your digestive system, respiratory system, pulmonary system, nervous system, reproductive system, and psychological systems.

Easier said than done, I know. You may sometimes feel over stimulated or super active. As an active person, I very often find myself just "doing stuff" and staying up late.

However, my body tells me that I neglect my sleep and relaxation. What happens next, is that I need to get my wellness back and recover. I find myself so tired that I can't carry on my active lifestyle. I have repeated this vicious cycle quite a few times until I finally learned my lesson. There is time for everything. Balance is the key. I don't want to use my health "credit card". Now, how about you? Do you know that the commission is high?

Now, in the evenings I get off-line and plan some gentle exercises like yoga or tai-chi (something I have gotten into only recently). I also read. In the evening, I try to go for shorter books because I know that I usually get so absorbed in a good read that I miss my bedtime. Yes! In other words, I got my body used to mental and physical activity in the morning and holistic relaxation in the afternoons and evenings.

- **Support networks.** It doesn't matter if it's our friends and family playing cheerleaders or online chat forums and message boards. As long as people support our work we are more inclined to stick with it. Make sure to tell those closest to you of your goals and aspirations. Join like-minded groups on your favorite social media sites and join community groups to exchange recipes. We are social creatures. We need to exchange our views, plans, and progress. We need people to support it no matter what we like to think about ourselves.

To be honest, I couldn't find any alkaline diet fans locally. Most of my friends thought I was going mad. This is why I decided to make some "alkaline buddies" on-line. I think it's really amazing that in this day and age you have the possibility to interact with people all over the globe and motivate one another. I take advantage of this opportunity every day, how about you?

Of course, don't go overboard. I know people who do much more research and are much more active in all those on-line groups and forums. Though at the end of the day they go against alkaline lifestyle. Why?

Because too much technology and on-line life is acidic. You need nature and oxygen on a daily basis.

- **Double up.** Often without conscious intent we will 'change' or alter, our food and beverage choices while in the presence of our friends and family to match theirs. If it is possible to avoid this, "recruit" them. The same goes for spouses, partners, children, roommates, or any others living in your homes. You don't have to bore them, lecture them or condescend them (these are all sure ways to end up fighting the battle all alone). Make them aware, try the "Did you know...""". But don't make them feel bad if they opt not to listen. This is your program after all

This is what I did: I committed myself to the *alkaline cooking challenge*. It was a *30 days challenge*. Every day I experimented with new recipes, or even took some traditional recipes. Like for example, Spanish paella. I tried to make them more alkaline by using quinoa instead of white rice and adding more green veggies and serving it with a big salad and avocado slices. I would try to cook something new every day and so I learned some great tricks. Then, I decided to throw a healthy party at my place. I invited a bunch of my friends over and they were just amazed.

Let me share this super alkaline Asian recipe, you can do the same for your family and friends, and you don't have to spend a month or more experimenting every day, I am giving you this ready and already-tested recipe that I know they will absolutely LOVE...

Ginger Quinoa Stir-fry

Serves:2-4

Ingredients:

- ½ squash of your choice (seeded and cubed 1")
- 2 stalks chopped celery
- 1 chopped green bell pepper seeded
- 1 whole sliced onion
- ½ inch grated ginger
- 3 minced garlic cloves
- ½ cabbage head of your choice
- 1 cup each: packed spinach and kale (chopped)
- 2 teaspoons crushed red pepper
- 4 Tablespoons coconut oil
- 3 Tablespoons Braggs liquid aminos
- 3 cups cooled cooked quinoa

Instructions:

1. Heat half of the coconut oil in a big frying pan. Fry onion, bell pepper and celery for 4 mins. Add ginger and garlic. Cook for one minute.
2. Put in the squash and fry for a few minutes until squash is tender.
3. Add about half of the Braggs and the seasonings along with the greens. Stir fry for a minute. Dump all into a bowl and set aside.
4. Heat the other half of the coconut oil in the same pan over medium high. Add quinoa and the rest of the liquid aminos. Stir fry until warm. Turn off heat and stir in vegetables. Enjoy!

If you eat out, one tip that I can give you is to toughen up. It's your life, your food and your choices. Search for healthy vegan or vegetarian restaurants. Even if you are not a vegan or vegetarian, you and your family or friends can try out something new. I love vegan places as they are so creative.

Family occasions, celebrations and work meetings (as well as Christmas dinners) very often include drinking alcohol. Alcohol is acid-forming. Here is my question for you: why do you drink first of all? Is it because you need to loosen up? Or is it because there is someone that you can't stand and you drink because of that feeling? For example, is there any annoying family member or a colleague?

You are not alone my friend.

We need to learn how to face certain individuals that we don't really want to spend time with. Simply take a few deep breaths and try to find at least one positive thing about that person, even if they are jerks. There must be something. Maybe they behave in certain way because they are facing some big problems. Maybe they are insecure?

You don't need to resort to alcohol. There are plenty of other healthy tools that can help you relax or loosen up (yoga, meditation, reiki, NLP, relaxing herbal infusions). First of all- work on your mindset. If you feel shy and drink to hide it, it's better to take action now and get to the root of the problem. You don't want to depend on alcohol all your life to "have a good time". I am not telling you not to have the occasional glass of wine (organic wine is good for you, of course, moderation is the key) or a cold beer in the summer (beer is extremely acidic and once you start going alkaline, beer might even be making you sick, tiny amounts of course, are fine, why not?).

Alcohol should be used and enjoyed in small amounts when we already feel happy. <u>Not because we want to feel happy.</u>

- **Celebrate dietary victories.** Set benchmarks such as one week of good behavior. For example: completing thirty minutes of exercise so many times a week, going for a walk around the block every night, engaging in physical activities with the kids for at least an hour a few nights a week, sticking to your diet for a certain period of time, etc. Treat yourself to a movie, the arcade, the mall, whatever makes you happy. Periodic rewards or acknowledgment are great tools of reinforcement and motivation. You are basically beginning a new cycle. For example, a 24 h challenge, a 7 days challenge, a 30 days challenge, or even a 100 day challenge. I do them twice a year, not only for health and fitness, but also for my career and personal life.

Go for a challenge- you will have something to look forward to after the challenge is completed (or a part of it is completed). I suggest it is something like a nice trip, catching up with friends, shopping for new clothes, getting a new haircut. Please remember not to indulge in any "acidic" kind of rewards. You know what I am talking about. We have already stated that the alkaline lifestyle is a deep change. So you can't just carry on to associate pleasure to unhealthy, acidic foods. Your body and mind deserve much more.

PART IV- ALKALINE AND HOLISTIC NUTRITION TIPS

Every year over two billion dollars are spent for both prescriptions and over-the-counter ways to prevent and control ailments such as heartburn, indigestion, and reflux. The beauty of the alkaline diet is in the emphasis on eradicating these problems through educated dietary choices. This is the real holistic approach.

You can easily get started today- simply by making some minor adjustments to your existing diet. Baby steps. I always try to make things simple and easy to apply. Once you apply it - you will feel the amazing benefits of Alkalinity and from there you will want to carry on.

The alkaline diet is not a diet but a lifestyle really. It encourages you to add more alkalizing foods and drinks into your diet so that your body can heal itself naturally. How?

Alkaline Diet Crash Course- Understand the Basics

The pH of most of our important cellular and other fluids (like blood) is actually designed to be at pH of 7.35 (slightly alkaline).

The body has an intricate system in place to always maintain that healthy, slightly alkaline pH level – no matter what you eat. This is an argument that many alkaline diet skeptics use and I get it. It's 100% true. This is not the goal of the alkaline diet. We just can't make our blood's pH more alkaline or "higher." Our body tries to work really hard for us to help us maintain our ideal pH (7.35). We can't have a pH of 8 or 10. If we did we would be dead.

The entire focus of the alkaline diet is to give your body the nourishment and healing tools it needs to MAINTAIN that optimal 7.35 pH almost effortlessly.

If we fail to do so, we torture our body with an incredible stress! Yes- when the body has to constantly work overtime to detoxify all the cells and maintain our pH it finally succumbs to disease. Then, it stops working for us and we end up in an over-acidic state.

Let me just name a few cases of what can happen if we constantly eat an acidic diet (also called SAD - Standard American Diet) that is not supporting our body at all. Our body ends up sick and tired of working overtime and may manifest one or more of the following conditions:

-constant inflammation

-immune and hormone imbalance

-lack of energy, mental fog

-yeast and candida overgrowth

-digestive damage

-weakened bones (our body is forced to pull minerals like magnesium and calcium from our bones in order to maintain alkaline balance it needs for constant healing processes).

In summary, eating more alkaline foods helps support our body so that it can work for us at optimal levels while eating more acidic food doesn't help at all. The alkaline diet is not about magically raising our pH but helping our body rebalance itself by supporting its natural healing functions.

However, it's not only about what we eat - it's also about how we live and what we think. It's not just a diet; it's a lifestyle. If you want vibrant health and alkaline wellness, try to be outdoors more, meditate, laugh, spend time with family and friends, do things you enjoy so that you can de-stress, practice mindfulness...It's not only about nutrition.

*Over the years, I have also learned that obsessing too much about food or health can be bad. I had to learn to let it go and focus on creating my healthy, alkaline lifestyle but at the same time **accepting occasional treats and cheats**. I had to learn to listen to my body and ignore some of the gurus' advice. You see - when you are too strict on yourself, this attitude takes away your emotional wellness. Balance is the key: we don't want to be too strict and too obsessed, but we don't want to end up being too lenient as well. You need to be honest with yourself and ask yourself what you can do better and reclaim responsibility for your health and wellness. It's always great to look for that next level, however it's also good to cultivate the sense of gratitude and accomplishment for what we have already managed to change in our diets and lifestyles.*

Oftentimes, it's not about eating less - but about eating right.

If you want to take care of your health and restore your energy levels and achieve your ideal weight, the general rule is to make 70%- 80% of your food alkaline, the rest can be acidic (still remember to go for quality and choose organic as much as you can, not all acidic foods are bad, we also need them in some small %).

Be sure to download your free Alkaline Wellness Toolkit (it includes recipes and charts) as well as other free gifts I have for you (including guided meditation and a free audiobook on mindfulness) from:
www.holisticwellnessproject.com
Simply visit www.holisticwellnessproject.com and go to "free stuff" section to get your free eBooks and audiobooks now.

Back to alkaline diet motivation and information. Simplicity is alkaline. It is our Western society that got used to "eat as much as you can" pattern and just mixes it all up. It is simply not good for your digestion and the more strain you put on your digestion the more tired you will feel. All oriental medicines, for example Ayurveda and TCM, employ Alkalinity in their own way. They stress the importance of proper digestion and encourage people to keep it simple. Make up your mind, make it "mindful". What are you going to have now? Is it really worth mixing it all up?

Alkalinity and good metabolism go hand in hand. Successful metabolism is defined as the proliferation and absorption of enzymatic minerals and vitamins. Potassium, calcium, and sodium drive the catalytic processes of cellular and nerve transmissions and give bones structure and rigidity. Magnesium contributes to and provides the energy for over three hundred reactions, plus oversees and regulates DNA synthesis. It provides and promotes efficient neuronal and nervous system firing and maintains blood glucose and pressure levels. But for our bodies to reap the benefits of our food we must first rid our bodies of any and all 'crap'. Or more specifically the particles and residues that are blocking absorption sites and preventing a cascade of bodily function.

TIP #1- Eliminate sugars, processed foods, and pre-packaged meals.

Being pressed for time seems to be the motto of the modern and contemporary culture. But it is killing us in multiple ways. Often the items consumed don't technically qualify as food, but usually they are the cheapest and the most advertised. Many of us don't have the time to look beyond this as we have been led to believe that health is expensive so it becomes a vicious cycle.

Prepackaged, or convenience foods, often hold no nutritional value with the worst offender often being high levels of sodium.

Sodium

Sodium is a mineral that our bodies rely upon. Therefore, most foods naturally have some. It is recommended that we get 2500 mg of sodium a day (National Institute of Health). This is enough to encourage successful metabolism while everything else is mainly for the sake of our taste buds. It is this excess amount that builds and becomes detrimental to proper cellular functioning. An abundance of sodium leaves us wanting more sodium, either in the forms of sodas or unhealthy, processed foods. Sodium dehydrates you. It encourages you to consume more products that are unnatural and foreign to the body. With nowhere to go they convert into fat.

Thanks to an increasing awareness of the ill effects of a sodium rich diet (obesity, bloating, high blood pressure, diabetes, heart disease, etc.) more products are being marketed as low-in sodium. Still, it is highly suggested that you read labels and

34

check serving sizes regardless of <u>what the front of the label says</u>. Be sure to note the serving size, this is located in small print under the heading.

So many foods are bought in the name of time management. It is our default thinking and the 'reasoning' for not buying fruits and vegetables. But the truth is that many foods, such as broccoli, spinach and zucchinis, take less time to cook than we spend waiting in the drive thru or a restaurant.

Nowadays, many foods can be bought cleaned, cut, and sliced. Diced fruit and salads can be bought bagged. To be honest, I am not a big fan of bagged salads, but they serve as my last resort tool when I am really pressed for time. They are much better than frozen pizza or lasagna! What I am more into doing is making sure I can always crunch on a healthy salad and don't overpay for bagged salads (if you only stick to those, it may come off a bit expensive in the long run). I get fresh spinach, kale, endives, lettuce and salads to wash them and chop them and store them in small containers in my fridge. This strategy allows no excuses. I have an alkaline, green "base" for my salads ready.

Another trick is to have my oils ready!

Herb Infused Alkaline Oils

I love olive oil and coconut oil, but sometimes I like to spice them up with some herbs. Garlic is super alkaline and it is a natural antibiotic, though many people overlook it. What I do is: I mix some olive oil with a couple of minced garlic cloves, some rosemary, thyme and sometimes even mint. I store the mix in glass jars or bottles. I have my healthy salad dressing ready to grab! So easy and so healthy! Moreover, this can be also done on the budget! Back to oils- make sure you pick up good quality cold-pressed oils. I usually use olive oil for my salads and coconut oil for stir-frying and baking.

Coconut Oil (good fats!)

- Coconut oil is also a great butter substitute. If you can't imagine your morning without toast, simply switch to healthy alternatives. Choose integral, gluten-free bread (it is OK in small amounts) and use coconut oil instead of butter.
- If you crave sugars, simply take 1 tablespoon of coconut oil. It usually does the trick for me!
- Coconut oil is an amazing cooking companion and makes your meals taste oriental and mysterious.
- It's also great on your body, hair and can be mixed with essential oils for a relaxing body massage.

Natural Remedies

Alkaline Lifestyle is a serious life transformation. If you really want to live in an alkaline way, I recommend you start exploring the world of natural remedies. Instead of looking for quick fixes and solutions in pills and medications it may be a good idea to substitute them with natural, holistic remedies that also aim to eliminate the cause of your sickness, not only the symptoms.

My mini disclaimer here- I am not saying that allopathic medications and allopathic medicine are useless. Quite on the contrary they can save lives. They are needed for "serious cases". However, they are very often abused. For example you have a headache, a backache, menstrual cramps or digestive problems and end up choosing quick fixes and forgetting about the amazing natural and holistic opportunities that are also alkaline. I can't provide the same recipe for everyone, but my general suggestion is that if you tend to suffer from any common (or uncommon) complaints, research the world of homeopathy and phytotherapy. A qualified homeopath, naturopathic doctor and phytotherapist can provide you with long-term and sustainable solutions. Homeopathy helped me treat uveitis, which is a serious eye condition related to the immune system and it can lead to blindness. This is why I am so passionate about sharing my message with the world.

Here are a few natural, alkaline tips:

- Menstrual cramps- massage your belly and lumbar area with fennel essential oil or basil essential oil, mint is also great (dilute in a good quality cold-pressed vegetable oil, use 5-10% concentrations for your blends). Don't apply undiluted. You can also try chamomile infusions and fish oil extracts.
- For relaxation, and/or tension headaches, try Melissa infusion or verbena/ valeriana infusion. It will also help you relax.
- Been working in your office all day? Go for a facial self-massage. Use 1 drop of verbena essential oil (don't sunbathe after using this one, it is phototoxic) or/ and mint oil in 1 teaspoon of your chosen vegetable oil (for example coconut oil). Massage your forehead (avoid eye, mouth and nose contact). Squeeze your eyebrows and the point between them (the "third eye"). Applying cucumber slices on your eyes, will help relax even more. No need to get a pill.

Anxiety, insomnia, headaches and stress can also be reduced by yoga, meditation and mindfulness. Try it now. Put the booklet down, sit down for about 15 minutes and breathe. Just breathe and BE. You will be alkalizing your body and mind. You can do it at work, just have a break, it can be even 5 minutes.

Remember that I have free audiobooks (mindfulness and meditation) that can help you. You can download them at:
www.holisticwellnessproject.com/subscribe-newsletter

Fruits and Veggies

Contrary to belief, your food bill will not skyrocket by buying fruits and veggies. Any differences will be minimal and ambiguous as quantity is also of issue and that is subjective. Often the best buys are found at farmers markets, roadside stands and produce markets. Any establishment that cuts out the "middle man" and offers food directly from the farm to the table will be cheaper. Check out local farms online, as many are certified Community Supported Agriculture. Also, CSA's offer monthly subscriptions for seasonal fruits that are delivered straight to your door. Some CSA subscriptions invite you out to the farm once a month to pick your own produce. If farms are not available to your area, frozen and canned vegetables are fine. Always buy the no-sodium added type if possible or rinse it off thoroughly with cold water for at least one minute to remove factory seasonings and salts.

Also, standing contrary to what we believe or like to believe, fruits and vegetables cook in minutes. They make quick and easy additions to salads, stews, soups and are equally nutritious frozen or fresh. We just have to reprogram, reset, orientate, and reformulate our default preconceptions and perspectives to include color.

★ Make a large salad, it will keep in a covered bowl for three days in your refrigerator (don't use salsas or oils if you want to keep it for later, use oils/salsa only before serving on separate plates). While you're at it, cut up containers of cucumbers, carrots, buy some raisins, almonds and an assortment or your favorite dried fruits. Then you can always have a variety of salads to choose from for lunch or dinner. Also, celery is a good quick inexpensive addition to any meal or snack. To break the monotony of plain celery try it with peanut butter, hummus, vegetable and onion dips.

I also encourage you to experiment with oils, herbs and spices. I recently came up with a really nice curry salad dressing: a bit of olive oil and curry powder plus minced garlic and Himalaya salt. So delicious and alkaline!

TIP #2 – Marinades

Marinades are a great way to bolster the flavor or to tenderize and even alkalinize acidic foods like fish, meat or tofu without additives or processed salts.

☆ tip-   Do not marinate fish longer than 20 minutes, as it will fall apart.

You can also marinate vegetables, for example peppers, zucchini and radish. These will be a nice addition to your raw food alkaline challenge and will bring a new variety of taste. If you think that tofu is boring, go ahead and marinate it. Use the same spices as you would use for your usual piece of meat.

- If possible, try for organic olive oils, some fruits, vegetables, and fresh herbs.
- Toast all nut additions. Also, try roasting veggies such as peppers and tomatoes. Just slice and space out on a baking tray. Cook for 10-12 minutes in a 425 degree

Fahrenheit or 220 degree Celsius oven. Since ovens vary times and degrees can also vary.

- If using dried herbs in a sauce or marinade let them sit in the mix unadulterated for 2-4 minutes. This allows the herbs to 'wake up' and diffuse.

TIP #3 – Snacks

Snacking can easily be our downfall, though we do need 'pick-me ups', we often confuse boredom with hunger. Now that we have decided to stick to mindful eating, we must be aware of those "*I am bored -I want to eat*" patterns as they are not supporting us in our healthy alkaline goals at all. To avoid this, try drinking a glass or two of water with lemon. Even better, fruit infused water since it fills the stomach. Some other simple snacks include:

- gluten-free wraps (filled with veggies or home-made marmalades)
- organic protein bars store bought or homemade
- celery sticks
- carrot sticks
- homemade tortilla chips (recipe in back)
- apple and pear pieces
- cucumber

The list above is just a few examples of things that can be snacks. Feel free to create your own. Have something ready to satisfy your sweet tooth as well (check out my recipes in the bonus chapter).

Foods such as apples and pears turn brown with exposure to oxygen. To help prevent this, cover them in lemon juice (It will also help alkalize them as most fruits, even though healthy and natural, are not really that alkaline).

Do the same with avocados (I love avocados by the way!). Avocadoes are one of the top alkaline foods ever and lemon/lime juice plus some herbs and oils will give it an amazing taste. In other words- use lime and lemon juice as much as you can. Spice up your water, salads and foods.

Don't be afraid to eat. Eat real foods. Fuel your body and mind with natural, alkaline foods. Go for raw foods as much as possible. Challenge yourself and go for quick, raw veggie snacks. Juice vegetables and make yourself delicious green smoothies. Focus on energy. Your alkaline bank account needs to maintain its positive balance, right?

★   For a quick and delicious snack, preheat the oven to 400 degrees Fahrenheit or 200 degrees Celsius, and cover a baking tray with either kale (I have already included the exact recipe) or spinach and drizzle it with olive oil. Feel free to experiment with cooking times, oven temperatures, and seasonings to find which works best for you. There are great substitutes for chips. Now you can snack without feeling guilty.

TIP #4 - Open your pores, drink more water, and sweat.

Sweating is great for detox. So help open those pores up. I recommend natural tee tree soap and sugar cane scrub. You can also use raw oats as a body scrub. Add drinking water into your day, always clean, filtered, quality water. Try to drink it as much and as often as possible. Add lemon and lime juice. Add some mint to spice it up. Our contemporary diets leave our bodies in a state of dehydration, so drink up! If you should find yourself the victim of water monotony, experiment with fruit and herb infused water...

Fruit Infused Spa Water

- Fruit infused spa water is natural and free from excess sugars, sodium's, additives, colors, and preservatives that sodas and flavored waters contain. Any noticeable additions can impart harmful constituents that can easily derail your hard work. Go for natural.

- The rule is very simple. In a jar, you mix some filtered water with a few pieces of your chosen fruits. I usually go for lemon and lime slices mixed with fruits like peaches, melons, apples and even bananas. I add mint or rosemary as well. If you are really pressed for time and want your fruit infused water to taste great as soon as possible, I suggest you stick with citrus fruits. They are really quick to infuse. For optimal results, I suggest you cover your jar and store it in a fridge for about 1 hour.

- Spice it up with some creative ice cubes- you can use fresh orange juice or lemon juice mixed with water and freeze it into ice cubes. I have recently gotten into experimenting with beet juice and I use it for ice cubes. The color effect that they have is just amazing, plus they are highly alkaline. Kids love creative ice cubes in fruit infused water and I have realized (I have a little nephew) that they may even become more interested in fruit infused spa water than artificial sodas and similar unhealthy drinks.

- You can store your fruit infused spa water in a fridge for about 24, even 48 hours. I always prefer to go for fresh though. I like to prepare it before I go to bed and enjoy it when I get up. I love it especially in the summer.

- A quick fix *on the go*- you just take a big glass, add a few lemon slices (add your chosen fruit slices as well), some fresh mint and a few ice cubes. Cover up for a few minutes and then drink. You can always re-fill the glass. Of course the flavor won't be that intense, but you can still hydrate your body and get more vitamins. Fruit infused water is all- natural vitamin water and a great naturopathic tool for weight loss, detox and revitalization.

You can learn more about Fruit Infused Water from my book:
"Fruit Infused Water: 50+ Original Fruit and Herb Infused SPA Water Recipes for Holistic Wellness, Detoxification, Weight Loss and High Energy Levels."
You can find it on my blog- HolisticWellnessProject.com or directly on Amazon.

MOVE YOUR BODY- IT'S ALKALINE

Adding exercise into your day is not to suggest that you become some kind of an 'endorphin junkie' and rush out and buy a bunch of machines or start training for a marathon(of course, I am here to support you if you are into a high water jump. I am a big fan of high water jumps!). It simply means to take the stairs instead of the elevator (or "the lift" as it is called outside of North America), opt for parking spaces that require a walk to the front door and everyday incorporate a little more of your street into a daily walk. Gather a group of friends or neighbors and go for a walk around the neighborhood, park, or a lake. Just move your body and you will be happier.

Get out in the back yard and play ball, tag, or fetch with your kids or pets. If you live in the right area walk to the store and reward yourself with a healthy smoothie when you get there. Ride your bike to the library to check out books on yoga and meditation. Be creative and incorporate some form of activity in your schedule and each day (or week or month) try to incorporate a little more. Treadmills, gyms, and saunas work too.

TIP #5 - Cut back/eliminate on sodas and coffee.

Coffee is a legal drug. You can have it anytime you want, which makes it easy to lose control and poison your body with toxins. People meet up to catch up over a cup of coffee. Offices offer free coffee to their employees. Some people can't even imagine their cup of coffee without a cigarette (by the way- cigarettes are extremely acidic and so are all drugs!).

I know that many of you can't imagine living without coffee, that's fine. Just use it occasionally and don't abuse it. Listen to your body.

Caffeine uses the same neural pathways as illegal substances to activate the reward/ pleasure centers in our brains. Many of the chemicals and additives are counterproductive for humans. Stimulants depress the active/reactive firing of our nervous systems to counter our perceptions so we slow down. They slowly break our systems down but leave us wanting more. The same mechanism goes for sugar, cocaine and other drugs. Yes, sugar is a drug, the same as cocaine and as some sources say, even more addictive.

But drinking natural, alkaline, caffeine-free drinks such as herbal teas can be a great option. You will think clearer, better, and faster. Create your own herbal tea rituals and enjoy them. You will find plenty of different tips and recipes on my blog: http://www.holisticwellnessproject.com/blog/alkaline-diet/

Also, remember to grab your free eBook:

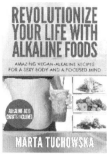

Download link:

While pre-packaged herbal teas are the most convenient, it is often a lot cheaper to make your own. Plus, you can control the amount of time the herb has to distribute itself throughout the tea. Fresh herbs such as ginger, thyme, oregano, parsley, lavender and turmeric make excellent herbal drinks both hot and cold. When purchasing pre-packaged teas make sure they don't contain any artificial flavors.

★ Example recipe- Boil 2 cups water. Be sure to add enough extra water to cover any evaporation. Once at a boil throw in 2 herbal tea bags, 3-4 peeled coin sized pieces of ginger or turmeric, or a handful of thyme, lavender, chamomile, parsley, or oregano on the stem. Let it sit and brew in the pot for 15-30 minutes. The longer it sits the stronger the infusion will be. The herbs are a great source of antioxidants that promote a strong and healthy immune system that eliminates harmful bacteria and free radicals. Many herbs also have antibiotic and anti-inflammatory properties that prompt vascular fluidity and health.

★ Try mixing various teas with fruit juices. Use alkaline, non-sugary fruits such as limes, lemons, grapefruits. You can also use apple or orange juice occasionally. For example thyme, mint, or lavender mix great with natural lemonade (water with fresh lemon juice). Mint and ginger can be paired with lime juice and grapefruit juice. Ginger and/or thyme can be infused into tomato juice. But try different concoctions and find out which ones best suit you. You can even make ginger juice...try it!

★   Fill up empty water bottles with tea and take it with you.

★   Green tea tastes great mixed with some fresh apple and grapefruit juice. I picked it up from my dad, he is a big fan of green tea. Ideally, the alkaline diet should be caffeine free and green tea is not considered alkaline. So if you want to make it strictly alkaline go only for caffeine /theine free natural herbal infusions. However, green tea is great to make this transition. It helped me quit coffee actually.

Teas made and brought from home will always provide more nutrition as those bought containing coloring and flavoring for the sake of increased sales.

If you really need your coffee make sure you choose good quality organic brand. Try some natural almond milk in coffee. Cow's milk is extremely acidic and so it makes things worse. Make your own alkaline "latte" with almond milk or coconut milk.

Try to make your coffee weaker and weaker every day. Skip it on some days and have some green tea instead. If you can do a week's challenge and eliminate coffee, you will get your energy back. Remember to add more green vegetable juices and smoothies. Use liquid chlorophyll in you water- you will find yourself nicely energized and you won't even need coffee.

My favorite natural teas include Kukicha and Roibos tea. The latter has an amazing natural sweet taste and is great with almond or rice milk. Coffee deprives your body of minerals, whereas Roibos provides you with them. Which option are you going to choose..?

TIP #5 - Refrain from alcohol.

Ok, I have briefly mentioned alcohol when talking about the "friends & family factor". If you must have a glass or two of red wine or maybe a beer, it is acceptable one night a week if followed by a return to detoxing beverages or participation in a detoxifying event.

Let's say that you got invited to your best friend's wedding. Drinking may be inevitable, unless of course, you define yourself as a teetotaler and stick to this definition (it might do the trick!). You must remember to keep in charge and make sure that you stick to 70/30 rule...yes! 70% of what you drink (or more!) should be water. I also recommend homeopathy remedy called Nux Vomica (30CH). You take a few granules before you go out and a few while at the party and the morning after. It will help you maintain an alkaline balance and help your body get rid of alcohol toxins. But hey, this is not a magical cure that allows you to drink as much as you want. Mind power and understanding why you drink are the most important part of this process.

TIP # 6 - Get raw; start juicing and drinking smoothies

-Raw fruits and vegetables are excellent sources of vitamins and minerals. Extracting the juices allows us to get them in their most potent forms in a quick and easy way.
-Juice vegetables as much as you can. You can add some fruits to taste, but don't juice sugary fruits. It's better to blend fruits and use them in smoothies, but I don't really recommend fruit juices- too much sugar (and no fiber), and on the alkaline diet,

we want to avoid sugar in all forms. To sum up- juices? Yes, but juice veggies and alkaline fruits (non-sugary). Other fruits? Yes, but eat them or blend them, don't juice them.
-To be safe it is best to wash all fruits and vegetables. So try this, submerge them for twenty minutes in a mix of table salt and lemon juice.

These drinks can be made to be higher in one vitamin or mineral based upon your dietary needs. For example, you can make a drink high in protein for a boost of energy before or after a workout. Because of the chemical ingredients and high sodium levels it is best for your health to stay away from chemical, mainstream sports drinks. Although, our cells do need to replenish electrolytes after fervent athletic activities or high levels of performance. Herbal teas and juices can be made prior to excursions to replenish our cells.

Easy Smoothie Recipes for Beginners:

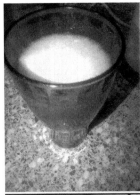

High Protein Smoothie
- A handful of kale
- 1 cup of coconut milk or almond milk
- A handful of Spinach
- ½ banana
- ½ cup of peach slices
- 1 tablespoon of coconut oil

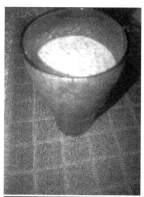

Breakfast Smoothie

- 1 cup almond milk or coconut milk
- 1/2 cup of strawberries or blueberries
- 1/2 cored & sliced apple
- 1/4 cup spinach
- Half avocado

If necessary add stevia for sweetness. Blend and enjoy!

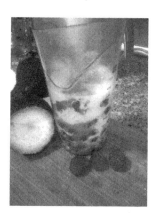

**Interested in Alkaline Smoothies and Juices?
Check out those free articles and learn more:
Juicing-**
www.holisticwellnessproject.com/blog/weight-
loss/alkaline-juicing-for-weight-loss/
Warm Alkaline Drinks-
www.holisticwellnessproject.com/blog/alkaline-
diet/warm-alkaline-drinks/
Smoothies-
www.holisticwellnessproject.com/blog/health-
wellness/super-energy-smoothies/

Coconut Water

Coconut water is miraculous! It is alkaline and helps your
body recover after strenuous workouts. You can also use it in
your smoothies to make them even more original and creative.

TIP #7 - Add herbs to your dishes.
Fresh is always best but some dishes do better with a more
subdued taste of dried herbs. Usually, the season, our location
or price determines if we use fresh or dried herbs. Eventually,
you will find that you like certain flavoring pairs. Fresh tends
to be stronger and more aromatic, but both versions hold
healthy properties when properly used. Generally, a teaspoon
more of dried herbs are required to achieve the same taste as a
pinch of fresh herbs. However, if possible taste before cooking.
Remember you can always add but you can't always subtract.

Herbs can be bought fresh in the produce section or dried in
the spice section. A lot of farms offer them as part of their
subscription plans, but they can also be grown at home,
indoors or outdoors, or in soils, pots, terrariums, and on

window sills. They are also popular at farmers markets and roadside produce stands.

TIP #8 - Never skip breakfast.

Breakfast sets us up to start the day off on the right foot. It not only allows us the energy to create a longer to-do list for the day, but lets us do it. Time and time again studies have shown the importance of this meal, but still we either skip it or skimp on it.

Somewhere along the line the idea that certain foods were a great way to start of the day. Thus, the Traditional Western breakfast revolves around foods central to starches, grease, and carbohydrates. These foods require copious amounts of energy and often conflicting forms of digestion resulting in mid-morning lethargy, reflux, bloat, or indigestion.

No worries, at the end of this book we will give you some nice recipes that are quick and easy, but give our bodies the protein that it needs for successful beginnings. So even if that means drinking our nutrition there is no longer any excuse for you to miss or skimp on breakfast. You can also download your free alkaline diet resources from holisticwellnessproject.com or email me at: info@holisticwellnessproject.com. I will make sure you get your alkaline friendly recipes for free.

TIP # 9 - Make use of the crockpot.

A crockpot is a quick and undemanding way to enjoy your food. Crock Pots are great for providing nutritious meals without the work. Just throw in your ingredients and it does the rest. The crock pot is perfect when you are working long hours or spending the day running errands.

While cooking times vary, many recipes can cook while you're at work or while you are asleep. Since it's cooking low and slow you don't have to be so worried about it burning.

Shopping Tips

- Download the grocery store app on your phone, tablet, or similar device and go over their flyer during breaks or lunch. Here you can search the entire store, certain department, items, prices, and get coupons.

- Plan the week's meals and snacks.

- Use the sale items (buy one get one free deals) to make the week's meals.

- Make meals in advance and store them in airtight containers in your freezer.

- Buy foods that can be used for multiple meals and snacks in one week. Don't fear leftovers or feel compelled to eat the entire thing. Recycle your food.

- Buy up to the limit of frozen goods. These items are staple foods and make excellent side dishes, casseroles, or ingredients for soups, stews, and salads.

- Look for sales on low sodium and minimally processed organic fruit juices, herbal teas, powdered teas and powders to mix in water for on the go. Don't be afraid to have fun and experiment. Play mad scientist: chemistry edition, and mix various flavors together so that you always have a diverse variety.

- The tying of herbs together is called a bouquet. Create a bouquet out of a package of fresh herbs bought in the produce section and drop it into a tea/juice mix. Bouquets also infuse flavor into soups, stews, gravies, salsas, and marinades.

- Contrary to assumption the intent of the alkaline diet is not to turn you into a vegetarian unless you want to go vegetarian; a healthy lifestyle is the goal. Meat is ok, just go for the lean varieties, such as chicken, fish, and turkey. Use 20/80 rule when creating your plate. Make sure you serve your chicken/fish or turkey with massive amounts of greens and you are fine to go. Personally, I recommend the vegan/vegetarian approach as much as possible but I don't want to preach to you. To sum up- you can go vegetarian but you don't have to. The choice is always yours.

Red meat should be eliminated or at least only used occasionally. You can do very well without it.

- Stores tend to inject chicken and ham with a high sodium broth. So always read the labels and any fine print on the packaging. Go for organic meat as well as look for vegan options as much as you can.

- From time to time herbs go on sale and depending on the herb it might be cheaper to buy the dried herbs and make your own tea bags. This can be achieved in several different ways. For instance, use a fine knife to cut a vertical slit underneath the string of a teabag and drop herbs into it then staple shut. Coffee filters make excellent tea bags, especially if you want to use fine dried herbs such as parsley. Just fold and staple the top shut or bring all of the open edges together and tie with string. Ziplock Baggies with small holes punched in it and all of the air removed can also be used. Be sure to check frequently though as sometimes not all of the air is removed and they float on top of the tea/water. Usually a push-pin is the best size for puncturing.

- When trying to strain liquids and the unwanted particles that are too fine to be caught, try pouring the liquid through a coffee filter. Mold it to the inside of your colander and catch those fragments. The cloth of a filter is porous enough to let the liquid through, but woven close enough to catch fine particles.

Shopping Tips part 2 - products you will need

- ***Green and alkaline powders and natural supplements-*** These are great to drink on the go or to drink in between meals for a 'pick me up'. Plus, both products can be used as the base ingredient for snacks such as granola bars, cookie/brownie bars and milk shakes. I especially recommend alfalfa powder- it is really alkaline and full of minerals. It is used in natural beauty treatments and will take care of your hair, nails and skin. I also like barley grass.

- ***Milk substitute-***Almond, rice, coconut, or even quinoa milk- the choice is yours. I also love coconut water in my smoothies.

- ***Salt substitutes and sweetener substitutes-*** Himalayan salt, sea salt, herbs, stevia are all excellent alternatives to excess sodium. It increases your urge to take carbonated beverages, excessively salty foods and other unhealthy habits.

- ***Oil substitutes-***Extra virgin olive oil, flaxseed, grape seed, or coconut oil are all viable alternatives.

- ***Tofu-*** Firm is the most recommended, as it is the easiest to handle and work with. Though you might find that certain flexibilities and textures work best with certain recipes. Remember to go for GMO-free, organic options.

- ***Sprouted, gluten-free tortillas and/or pita bread-*** these are excellent for green wraps. You can also use kale leaves to make it more alkaline.

- ***Hummus-*** Excellent dip or mayonnaise like addition to wraps and sandwiches. Chickpeas are not super alkaline, but they are not that acidic either. Soak chickpeas overnight. Boil them and blend them with fresh lime juice, olive oil and garlic. So yummy as a dip! I love it with carrots, kale or cucumber. If you can't tolerate legumes, go for veggie hummus. Zucchini hummus is one of my favorite choices. Add some tahini and you have a nutritious raw meal.

- ***Bragg Liquid Aminos-*** Great addition to foods to add a salty flavor without the extra sodium. Also, a great way to get more amino acids into your body. This is a great alternative to soy sauce (soy sauce is not alkaline).

- ***Nuts-*** Cashews, almonds, flaxseed, soy nuts, pumpkin seeds, sunflower seeds all make excellent snacks and are a unique, crunchy, healthy flavorful addition to mediocre dishes. Almonds should deserve particular attention here as they are super alkaline.

All of these products can be found in grocery stores, retail stores and health food stores. While this may sound absurd or even somewhat unrealistic and "too expensive", just remember that you do not have to buy all of these things at once. Also, a lot of the foods you have at home may be suitable to serve as ingredients in dishes or snacks.

Many websites and health food stores try to sell you vitamins and supplements.
I believe that one does not need to use all those supplements. One that works for you may be enough. In case of supplements, even natural ones, I suggest you consult your physician first. Maybe you don't need them really? Also be sure to pick a credible brand. Remember- first of all you need a balanced diet. You cannot fix a crappy diet by consuming massive amounts of supplements. Once your diet is healthy and balanced, natural supplements such as alkaline green powders or alkaline salts can take it to a whole new level- but do not expect miracles if you neglect your nutrition.

Additional Resources, Recipes + More Information
->Alkaline Cooking for Busy People:
www.holisticwellnessproject.com/blog/alkaline-diet/alkaline-lifestyle-for-busy-people/

->Mindful Eating:
www.holisticwellnessproject.com/blog/mindfulness/mindfulness-motivation-success/

->Quinoa and Quinoa Recipes:
www.holisticwellnessproject.com/blog/health-wellness/health-benefits-of-quinoa/

->Alkaline Supplements- Benefits and Recommendations:
HolisticWellnessProject.com

PART V: BONUS CHAPTER - ALKALINE RECIPES

Below are some recipes for quick and easy meals, snacks, and beverages. While I do hope that you enjoy them, the main purposes behind them are to serve as templates and guides for successfully bringing this diet into your day despite your schedule. I also want you to learn to be creative and start adding more fresh alkaline foods while eliminating acidic ones.

Beverages

Recipe#1.Lemon-Thyme-Tea

Serves- 8
Ingredients:

- Alkaline lemonade: 2 cups of water with fresh lemon juice of 2 lemons and 2 tablespoons of raw honey or maple syrup or a few drops of stevia
- 4-6 cups thyme tea

Instructions:

1. Pour the tea into the container with the lemonade, shake well, and enjoy.
2. Sweeten to taste if necessary with stevia, if more thyme is needed make a bouquet.
3. Tie together four or five sets of stems and leaves and drop that into the container.

4. The strings of tea bags are excellent for tying together herbs. While no special knot is needed, make sure it is adequately tied to keep it from coming apart.
5. Enjoy!

*Thyme is an excellent natural remedy for digestion and cold prevention. It is also extremely refreshing. This is my favorite "alkaline herbal lemonade".

Recipe#2 Apple Tea

Serves-2, 3 cups
Ingredients:

- Half liter of thyme tea
- 1/2 cup fresh green apple slices
- 1 tablespoon cherry juice or raw honey or a few drops of stevia

Instructions:

1. Brew thyme tea and cool down
2. Juice a few green apples to obtain fresh apple juice. You can also squeeze in a lemon or a grapefruit.
3. Mix thyme tea and apple juice in a jar. Add a few ice cubes.
4. Garnish with mint and lime slices.

Variations: This recipe is easy to use as a template for trying new herb/juice combinations. For example, try parsley instead of thyme and lime juice instead of apple juice.

Recipe #3 Chamomile-Ginger Tea

Serves- 4, 5 cups
Ingredients:

- 3-4 ^{chamomile} tea bags or put chamomile leaves in 1 liter of boiling water
- Stevia to sweeten
- 5 cups water
- 2 teaspoons grated and peeled fresh ginger
- ⅓ cup lemon juice

Instructions:

1. Prepare chamomile infusion and let it cool down. Add a few ice cubes to speed it up.
2. In the meantime, squeeze a few lemons for lemon juice.
3. Mix together in a jar and spice it up with grated ginger.
4. This is an excellent detox and anti-flu remedy. Drink to your heart's content.

Recipe#4 Pineapple-Oregano Tea (Anti-cellulite!)

Serves- 3 cups
Ingredients:

- Half liter of oregano tea (use 3 teabags or portions for 3 cups)
- Fresh juice of 1 grapefruit and lemon

Instructions:

1. Prepare oregano tea and let it cool down.
2. Squeeze 1 grapefruit and lemon.
3. Mix the ingredients in a glass jar. Add a few ice cubes.
4. Garnish with a slice of pineapple. You can also use a few pineapple chunks and infuse them.

This recipe is great for those who want to keep cellulite at bay. Make sure you drink 1-2 cups a day.

Recipe#5 Purple Horizon- Sweet Dreams!

Serves- 2 cups
Ingredients:

- 2 cups of water
- 1 tablespoon lavender
- 4-5 leaves of mint
- 1 tea bag chamomile
- stevia (optional)

Instructions:

1. Mix lavender and mint in 1 cup of water. Cover. Let infuse for 30 minutes.
2. In the meantime, prepare chamomile infusion (1 cup of water + 1 teabag).
3. Let it cool down.
4. Mix chamomile infusion with herb infused water from step 1.
5. Enjoy!

Recipe #6 Pick-Me-Up Sweet Treat!

This recipe will satisfy your sweet tooth...

Serves-2
Ingredients:

- 1 container vegan yogurt
- 2 teaspoons natural vanilla extract
- 1 apple
- 1 pear
- ½ cup strawberries
- 1 lemon
- Half cup of coconut water or almond milk

Instructions:

1. Blend the fruits with coconut water or almond milk (you can also mix two, why not?).
2. Place in a big glass. Add yogurt and vanilla extract on top, so delicious!
3. Serve cold for extra refreshment.

Recipe #7 Berried Pleasure!

Serves- 1
Ingredients:

- 1 tablespoon cocoa
- Half cup of baby spinach
- 1 cup of coconut yoghurt
- 1 cup assorted berries (strawberry, blueberry, etc.)
- 1 tablespoon coconut oil
- 1 cup of fresh grapefruit or lemon juice

Instructions:

1. Blend all the ingredients. You can also throw in some ice cubes.
2. Serve cold and garnish with fresh lime slices.
3. Enjoy, I do!

Recipe #8 Chocolate Bars Natural Cheat Day

Serves-2
Ingredients:

- 1 tablespoon chocolate protein powder or cocoa
- 3 protein bars with nuts and chocolate
- 1 avocado
- 1 cup of sweet almond milk
- A few strawberries (optional)
- 2 teaspoons of alfalfa powder
- 1 teaspoon of chlorella powder

Instructions:

1. Before placing all of the ingredients into a blender, chop the protein bars into slices to make for easier and more thorough blending.
2. Blend all the ingredients.
3. Stir well and cool down.
4. Garnish with some fresh mint leaves.
5. Enjoy!

Recipe #9 Lucky Green Charms

Serves-2
Ingredients:

- 2 cups kale
- 2 medium sized carrots
- 2 heads of broccoli
- Lemons, peeled
- 2 pears
- 1 apple
- 2 bananas
- 3 stalks of celery
- 2 cups of cooled green tea

Instructions:

1. Prepare 2 cups of green tea and let it cool down.
2. In the meantime, wash, peel and chop other ingredients.
3. In blender, blend adding green tea.
4. Serve immediately.
5. Enjoy!

This is a great recipe for those who need a tiny bit of theine in their smoothies. Do you want to quit/reduce coffee? Try this almost alkaline drink!

Recipe #10 Random Mix

This is what my blender and I created the other day and we feel like sharing it...

Serves: 2-3
Ingredients:

- 1/2 cup spinach
- 1 slice of watermelon
- 1 apple
- 1/2 banana
- 1 pear
- ⅓ cup grapes
- 1 tablespoon of alfalfa powder
- 2 cups of almond milk

Instructions:

1. Mix all the ingredients in a blender.
2. Add alfalfa powder and stir well.
3. Optional: sprinkle over some cinnamon.

Recipe #11 Proteini Naturale

Serves-2
Ingredients:

- 1 avocado
- ½ cup spinach
- 1 apple
- 1 pear
- ½ banana
- Juice of 1 grapefruit and 1 lemon
- Half cup coconut milk

Instructions:

1. Blend and enjoy!

Breakfast

Recipe #12 Tofu Mixer

Serves-2, 3
Ingredients:

- 2 cups crumbled tofu
- 2 cups of diced shallot, peppers, tomatoes, and celery
- 1 teaspoon basil
- Olive oil or coconut oil
- Himalaya Salt
- 1 garlic clove, minced

Instructions:

1. In a pot, pour 1 to 2 teaspoons of olive oil
2. Brown tofu with garlic for a few minutes.
3. Add peppers, tomatoes, and celery. Stir fry for a few minutes.
4. Empty onto plate and drizzle basil over dish, or season to taste.

Recipe #13 Tofu Wraps

Serves- 1, 2
Ingredients:

- 1 cup of crumbled tofu
- 1 teaspoon diced shallot
- 1 cup spinach/lettuce or kale
- 1 teaspoon almonds, cashews or pine nuts
- 1 cucumber
- 1 chopped or diced tomato
- pinch of turmeric, parsley, or oregano

Instructions:

1. In a pot pour 1 to 2 teaspoons of olive oil and brown tofu, shallot, spinach and nuts.
2. Empty into wrap and then top with cucumber, tomato, and herbs.
3. Enjoy, this is a really powerful breakfast!
   Who said that the Alkaline Diet is about going hungry..?

Recipe #14 Oatmeal and Fruit

A quick and easy protein laden and tasty way to start the day is some old fashion oats topped with fruit...

Serves-1
Ingredients:
Honey Oats

- 1 bowl old fashion oats (organic, unprocessed, I suggest Scottish oats)
- 1 sliced peach
- A few almonds
- Optional: Raw organic honey (1 tablespoon) /maple syrup or a few drops of stevia

Instructions:

1. Cook oats accordingly, slice peach over them to collect any falling juices.
2. Top with almonds and cover in organic honey or maple syrup.
3. Oats are high in protein so make an excellent choice for morning fuel, but it's even better if coupled with a protein smoothie or juice.

Recipe #15 Crockpot Oats

Serves-2, 3
Ingredients:

- 2 cups oats- old fashioned
- 6 cups of water
- 1 cup almond milk
- Optional: raisins and cinnamon

Instructions:

1. Cook on low overnight, 8 hours. The trick to this recipe is making sure your crockpot is halfway to ¾ full when starting to cook.
2. Due to differences in sizes this may mean more or less cups of water than the recipe calls for. Also, many will add more oats as to have more for the week ahead.
3. Store leftovers covered in refrigerator, add almond milk, or almond butter, and heat up if you wish.
4. Top with your favorite toppings.

Meals and side dishes

Recipe #16 Tofu Stir Fry

Serves-1 -2
Ingredients:

- 1 tablespoon olive oil
- 2 cups brown rice or quinoa
- 4 cups water
- ½ cup broccoli, carrots, and onion
- 2 cups of diced tofu, lightly cooked
- Seasonings or herbs to taste such as celery salt, table blend, etc.

Instructions:

This recipe can be cooked on either the stove top or Crock Pot. If using stove:
1. Heat oil over med-high heat, pour in rice and water.
2. Cook rice, constantly stirring it over medium-high heat.
3. Turn heat down to medium and add broccoli, carrots, and onion.
4. Cook 2 minutes and add tofu.

If using Crock Pot:

1. Put a mix of oil on the bottom and put rice on top of that.
2. Pour in enough water to fully cover rice.
3. Put the rest of the ingredients and the seasoning in.
4. Cook on low 4 hrs.
5. This dish is excellent on its own or it is great to pair with fish or more vegetables.

Recipe #17 Chicken Wrap

While not strictly alkaline, this is a great transition recipe for those who don't know where to start.

Serves-2
Ingredients:

- 1 tablespoon olive oil
- chopped or shredded chicken (2 cups)
- 3 trees broccoli
- 2 big tomatoes
- spinach or kale
- crumbled tofu drizzle with lemon juice
- ½ stalk of celery or 2 teaspoon of celery salt
- ½ teaspoon or torn up basil leaves (optional)

Instructions:

1. Let olive oil warm over medium heat.
2. Crumble tofu as putting in pot, lightly brown it.
3. Add chicken, spinach or kale, broccoli, tomato, and celery, constantly stirring until sufficiently warm and then empty contents into wrap and drizzle with lemon juice.

These can be made in advance and used for lunches and snacks for up to three days if kept refrigerated in an air container or package.

This recipe is also flexible if you are a vegetarian. Simply skip chicken and add more tofu.

Recipe #18 Kale Salad- Super Alkaline Power

Serves-3,4
Instructions:

- 2 cups Chinese cabbage
- 4-6 cups kale leaves
- ½ diced cantaloupe
- ½ honeydew melon
- 1 diced cucumber
- 1 tablespoon pine nuts although almonds, pistachios, or cashews make good substitutes
- ¼ cup bell peppers*
- olive oil
- basil
- ginger

Instructions:

1. Mix kale, nuts, and peppers in bowl then spread out on baking sheet.
2. Drizzle with olive oil.
3. Cook approximately 8-10 minutes.
4. Let cool and place back into bowl where all ingredients are mixed together.
5. Drizzle again with olive oil, add basil leaves and finely diced ginger.

* - Bell peppers tastes the same regardless of color. Differences in color only reflect a difference in the seeds and the time spent in the soil, but nothing else. So the color of the peppers should accommodate the dish.

Recipe # 19Veggi Pizza

Victory food to celebrate your dietary accomplishments without totally ruining your win.

Serves-2
Ingredients:

- 1 package homemade dough
- Crumbled tofu (1 cup)
- ½ cups mixed bell peppers
- 2-3 tablespoons spinach
- 1 cup mushrooms
- minced garlic, onion, and ginger
- 1 teaspoon each of basil, oregano, and parsley

Instructions:

1. Make dough according to package directions; to add to the taste cover it in some olive oil.
2. Mix pepper strips, spinach and mushrooms together in a bowl.
3. Mix basil, oregano and parsley together in a separate bowl.
4. Flatten dough to equal thin crust thickness.
5. Sprinkle with tofu.
6. Mix garlic, onion, ginger and let 'rain' on tofu;
7. Layer with pepper mix and top with herb mix.

Snacks

These are healthy and nutritious snacks that your body really deserves. All you need to do is it get rid of anything else (here I refer to foods that prevent you from being successful) so that there is no temptation. Make sure your kitchen is well equipped with healthy alternatives. No excuses...

Recipe #20 Squirrel Chow Alkaline Neutral Snack

Serves-2
Ingredients:

- ¼ cup pine nuts, soy nuts, almonds, and cashews
- ¼ cup sunflower seeds
- 1/4 cup raisins
- ¼ cup dried cranberries
- 1 cup of almond milk or rice milk

Instructions:

1. Mix ingredients together and you have an easy on-the-go snack.
2. Enjoy!

Recipe #21 Apple Berry Drink

Serves-2
Ingredients:

- ½ cup strawberries
- 1 apple
- Half cup coconut milk
- ¼ cup dried pomegranate or cranberries
- Juice of 1 grapefruit

Instructions:

1. Blend well and add some cinnamon to spice up.
2. Add some water for desired consistency if you wish.
3. Enjoy!

Recipe #22 Tortilla chips

Before you start-Pre heat oven to 400 Fahrenheit or 200 degrees Celsius

Serves-2
Ingredients:

- 5 gluten-free tortilla wraps
- olive oil to spray or drizzle
- garlic powder

Instructions:

1. Cut tortillas into triangles (the shape of the standard tortilla chip) and spread out on baking sheet.
2. Spray or drizzle with olive oil and sprinkle with garlic powder.
3. Cook for 8-10 minutes and serve with some raw vegetables.

Soups/Stews/Sauces

Recipe #23 Tofuni Dip
Serves-2
Ingredients:

- 1 cup of chopped tofu
- ½ chopped sweet onions
- 1 tablespoon minced garlic
- ½ cup garbanzo beans or cannellini beans
- juice of one lemon
- ½ teaspoon basil
- ½ teaspoon pine nuts

Instructions:

1. Sauté onion and garlic over medium heat.
2. Make sure tofu is dry before crumbling into blender or food processor.
3. Blend tofu, beans, onion, and garlic.
4. Stir in lemon juice and basil.
5. Put in a bowl and top with pine nuts.

Recipe #24Veggie Stew for the Crock Pot
Serves-2
Ingredients:

- 1 tablespoon olive oil
- 4 cups vegetable broth
- ⅓ cup diced carrots
- ⅓ cup spinach
- ½ corn
- ½ cup diced potatoes
- ½ cup mix of onion, garlic, and ginger
- 1 diced stalk of celery
- 3 teaspoons herb de Provence (Italian seasonings, equal parts basil, oregano, parsley, thyme, and rosemary)
- 2 teaspoons cumin
- pinch of turmeric

Instructions:

1. Make broth in pot on top of olive oil.
2. Add prepared ingredients to broth and top with seasoning.
3. Cook 8 hours on high, 10-11 hours if on low.

For more Alkaline Recipes check out The Alkaline Diet Lifestyle Cookbook 3 in 1 BOX SET (available in kindle and paperback for your convenience)

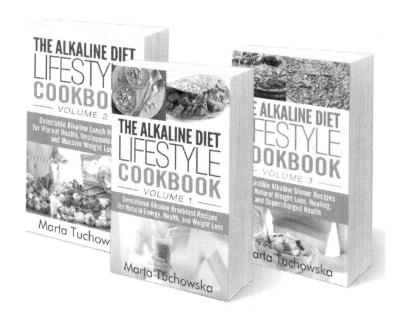

www.amazon.com/author/mtuchowska

CONCLUSION- YOUR HOMEWORK

We are now approaching the end of this book. I hope that you have managed to find at least one motivational and/or nutritional tip that can help you in your wellness endeavors. Your weight loss, wellness and health journey may start here. Alkalinity is sustainable. We are not taking about a fad diet here. However, this book was merely the first class. Since I am a really strict and demanding teacher, I have some homework for you...

Don't put it off. You know what it's like with homework that you don't want to do and then it's Sunday evening and you feel stressed out? I hope it will not be your case.

Don't wait till Sunday evening. Do it now. Start from healthy shopping first. Prepare yourself and your goals. Make Alkalinity your lifestyle. You will really enjoy it, I know you will!

Remember to download your free eBook at: www.holisticwellnessproject.com/alkaline-diet-ebook/giveaway.html

These are your new friends:

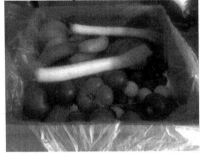

You have just learned the most important lesson: motivation, inspiration, dedication and preparation, as well as perseverance. You have passed the theory with flying colors, but now it's time to face the practical test. I am confident that you will score 100%!

If you enjoyed my book, it would be greatly appreciated if you left a review so others can receive the same benefits you have. Your review can help other people take this important step to take care of their health and inspire them to start a new chapter in their lives. At the same time, you can help me serve you and all my other readers even more.

I'd be thrilled to hear from you. As long as I know what you like, I can create more amazing recipes and tips that will help you on your journey.

I know you are busy and I would like to thank you in advance for considering taking a couple of minutes to review this book. Even 1 sentence will do!

ADDITIONAL RESOURCES FOR ALKALINE WELLNESS MOTIVATION

Looking for more recipes and wellness?

Follow me on Instagram and discover my holistic lifestyle secrets + dozens of alkaline recipes, picks and motivational videos that will help you keep on track throughout the day:

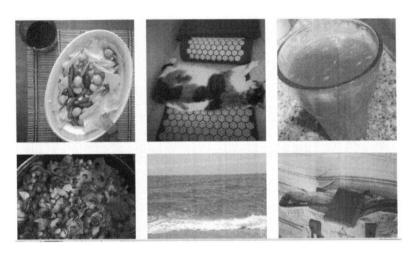

www.instagram.com/Marta_Wellness

Let Me Help You

If you have any questions, doubts, or you find my instructions confusing and need more guidance, please e-mail me. I am here to help. Don't be shy. I am also looking for feedback. If you have any suggestions that can help me improve my work, please let me know and I will take an immediate action to serve you better in the next editions. Thanks and have a fantastic day!

info@holisticwellnessproject.com

FINALLY- LET'S KEEP IN TOUCH

www.instagram.com/Marta_Wellness

www.facebook.com/HolisticWellnessProject

www.twitter.com/Marta_Wellness

www.pinterest.com/martaWellness/

www.udemy.com/u/martatuchowska

www.linkedin.com/in/martatuchowska

www.plus.google.com/+MartaTuchowska

43525347R00050

Made in the USA
San Bernardino, CA
20 December 2016